the pocket book of
sensational
orgasms

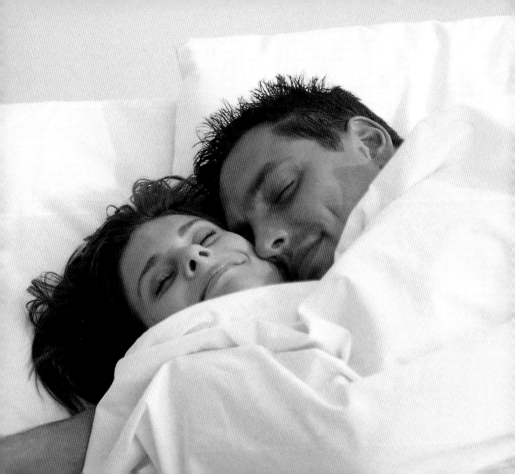

the pocket book of
sensational
orgasms

Richard Craze

Hunter
House
PUBLISHERS

For further information, please contact:
Hunter House Inc., Publishers
P.O. Box 2914, Alameda CA 94501-0914

Designed for Godsfield Press by *The Bridgewater Book Company*

Studio photography by *Alistair Hughes*
Illustrations by *Coral Mula*

Library of Congress CIP data is available

ISBN 0–89793–375–3 (pb)

Printed in Hong Kong

ORDERING INFORMATION
Trade bookstores and wholesalers in the U.S. and Canada, please contact Publishers Group West
Tel: 1-800-788-3213 Fax: (510) 528 3444

Hunter House books are available for bulk sales at discounts to qualifying community and health-care organizations.
For details, please contact: Special Sales Department
Hunter House Inc., P.O. Box 2914, Alameda CA 94501–0914

Tel: (510) 865 5282 Fax: (510) 865 4295
e-mail: ordering@hunterhouse.com

Individuals can order our books from most bookstores, by calling **(800) 266-5592**,
or from our website at **www.hunterhouse.com**

9 8 7 6 5 4 3 2 1 First Edition 02 03 04 05 06

Contents

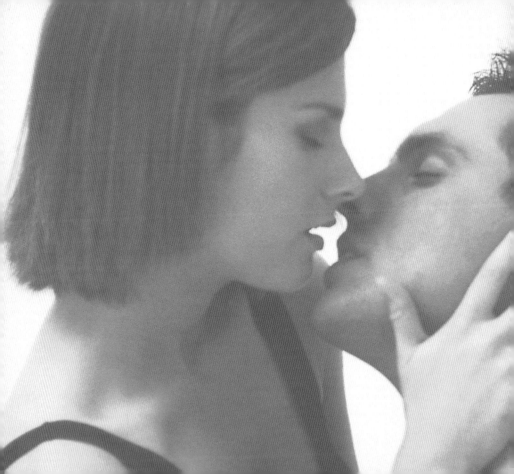

Introduction

The Pocket Book of Sensational Orgasms *is the perfect guide for people in a loving and stable relationship, because love and stability are the basis for great lovemaking. Making love can strengthen a relationship, and it is one of the most pleasurable experiences in life.*

The act of lovemaking has many stages, each of which is wonderful in its own way—but lovemaking becomes really special when it ends in a sensational orgasm. This book can help you and your partner enhance your lovemaking so that you will both enjoy heartstopping orgasms.

The first section of the book explains how and why orgasms take place, while the second gives you ideas on setting the scene for lovemaking and on how to arouse each other. We start with practical exercises for you to share together, explaining fantastic techniques to help you bring one another to orgasm—and for reaching orgasm together. And remember, practice really does make perfect.

Lovemaking and the Importance of Orgasm

To make love physically is literally to create love. When you make love with a partner for whom you care deeply and who cares deeply for you, you are strengthening the bond between yourselves, and expressing your mutual love and attraction in the most personal way possible.

PARTNERS IN A stable, loving, and committed relationship have a genuine desire to give each other as much pleasure as possible when making love—and a great way to demonstrate your care and consideration is to give each other really sensational orgasms.

Orgasms are important. They are not only an expression of love, but because bringing each other to orgasm is such an incredibly intimate act, one based on trust and understanding, orgasms are also spiritually rewarding—there is nothing quite like that amazing moment when you are at one with your partner on all levels.

Enhancing orgasms and turning them into something truly heartstopping takes a little time, a lot of practice, and clear, uninhibited communication. To make your lovemaking really sensational, commitment is needed from both partners—if you don't share the same enthusiasm, it's a lot more difficult to make it work properly.

Sharing this book is an ideal way to start. Read it together, and discuss what appeals to you and what doesn't. Try to keep an open mind—you may discover that something that puts you off at first is the very thing that ends up making the difference!

RIGHT *Making love when you are in a stable and committed relationship is a physical celebration of an emotional union that can greatly enhance your relationship.*

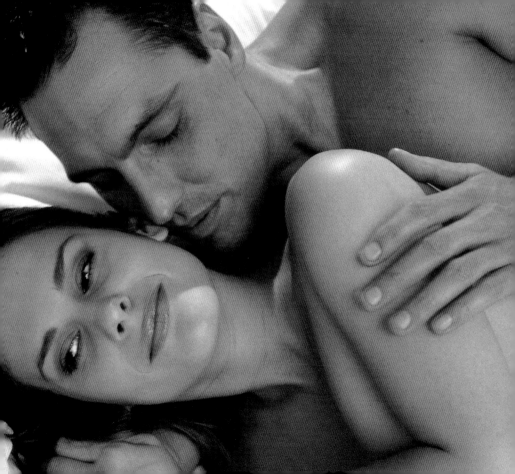

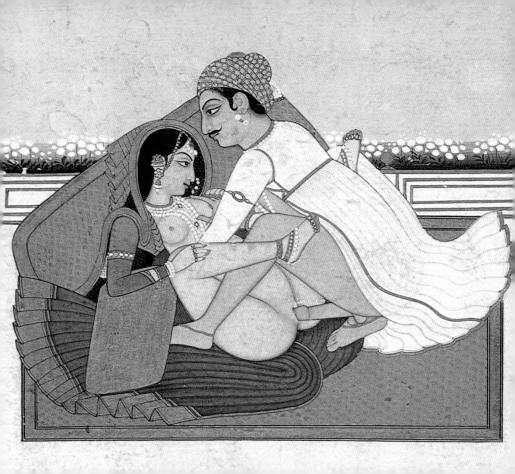

Orgasm in the 21st Century

Eastern cultures have always had a very positive approach to lovemaking. The ancient Chinese Taoist masters, for example, viewed sex as an essential exchange of yin and yang energy. Woman's yin essence (vaginal secretions) was believed to nurture man's yang essence (semen), so it was not only vital that lovemaking lasted as long as possible, so that the man received the maximum amount of yin essence, but also that the woman came frequently to orgasm, to ensure a plentiful supply of yin essence was maintained.

I N T H E W E S T, however, lovemaking has tended to be a rather taboo subject. Until very recently it was seen as a duty to be endured by women for the procreation of children and to satisfy men's drunken desires on a Saturday night—under the bedcovers and with the lights off! It certainly wasn't to be enjoyed by women—at least, not overtly. While the Eastern writers produced explicit books on the subject, such as the second-century Hindu classic, the *Kama Sutra*; in the

LEFT *An illustration from the* Kama Sutra, *an Indian erotic manual on the art of love.*

West, books such as D. H. Lawrence's *Lady Chatterley's Lover* were banned even in the progressive 20th century.

Fortunately, all that has changed now. The importance of women's orgasms has been recognized, and even men are encouraged to try multiple orgasms. Women in films are seen not only responding to lovemaking, but also frequently initiating it, and nudity is commonplace. Couples with sexual problems can get help from counselors. We can read about women's orgasms, watch them, and talk about them. The orgasm has come of age.

Why We Orgasm

The word "orgasm" comes from the Greek orgasmos, which means to swell or be lustful.
Why do we orgasm? The main reason, of course, is associated with the basic purpose of sex—
to procreate. A man's orgasm coincides with the ejaculation of semen into the woman's vagina,
and, if she is ovulating at the time, she may become pregnant.

THE MORE OFTEN lovemaking takes place during the ovulation period, the higher the chances are of conceiving—as long as the lovemaking results in male orgasm. Most of the time, however, we don't make love with the aim of making babies!

Unlike animals, who only mate when the female is fertile, we have discovered that to have an orgasm is an intensely pleasurable experience for both men and women, and that we can enjoy that experience whenever we like. By using contraceptives, we can give and receive pleasure through full intercourse without producing offspring, and by mutual masturbation we can give and receive the same pleasure without any danger that a pregnancy will result.

Although making love doesn't necessarily have to end in orgasm, it is the orgasm that marks the climax of lovemaking and provides the release of the tension that sexual activity produces. You will know that you are giving your partner sexual satisfaction when he or she has a sensational orgasm. In an intimate loving relationship, giving your partner this fantastic experience is equally as rewarding as receiving a sensational orgasm yourself.

RIGHT *Bringing each other to orgasm completes the act of love by producing a wonderful feeling of relaxation.*

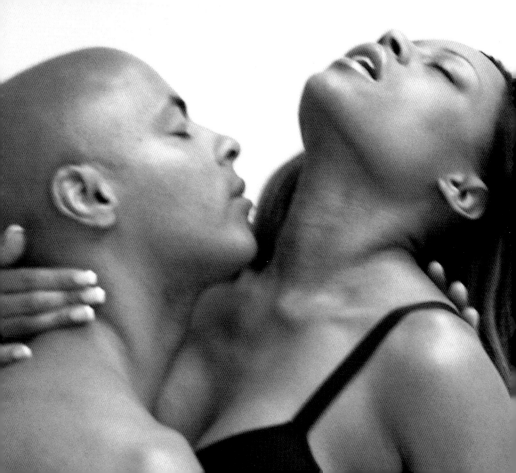

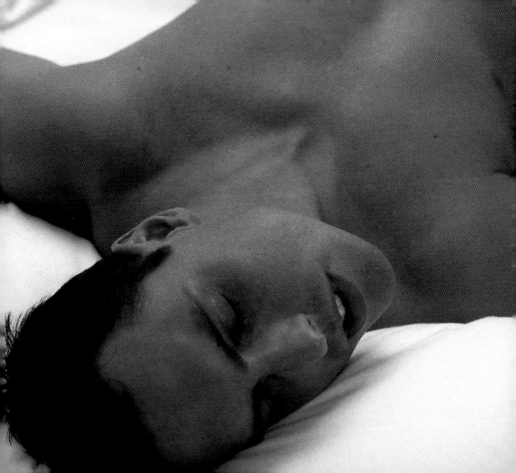

How We Orgasm

Men and women orgasm differently—but not that differently. It used to be thought that men and women needed different techniques—that a woman needed much more stimulation and that a man could achieve orgasm much more easily. Modern research has shown this to be untrue—achieving orgasm can be easy or complicated for both men and women.

WOMEN MASTURBATING on their own can achieve orgasm just as quickly as men masturbating. If a woman experiences delay in reaching orgasm when making love with a partner, it is only because her partner has not identified the best way to make it happen—that is why communication and practice are so important. A woman in the hands of a partner who knows how she likes to come will orgasm as easily as if she were masturbating herself.

So what happens when we orgasm? Technically, orgasm is an explosive discharge

LEFT *Orgasms are felt throughout the body, and can produce a feeling of temporary unconsciousness.*

of accumulated neuromuscular tensions, usually accompanied by groaning, a loss of physical control, rigidity throughout the whole body, an increase in heart and breathing rates, genital throbbing, and a loss of feeling or numbness in other parts of the body. Men will usually find their orgasm accompanied by ejaculation, and women may have an increase in vaginal secretions. If the orgasm is very intense, there may even be a sort of temporary unconsciousness—a wonderful sensation that you've floated away to a higher plane, similar to the sensations of spiritual orgasm described in the ancient Indian art of Tantric lovemaking.

All About the Female Orgasm

Some people used to believe that the only way a woman could have an orgasm was by having her husband make love to her in the missionary position, and if orgasm didn't happen, it was simply because she wasn't capable. And nice girls certainly didn't masturbate! However, those days are behind us, and we now know that women can enjoy intense, multiple orgasms.

BOTH WOMEN and men go through four phases in orgasm: excitement, plateau, orgasm, and resolution. In each of these phases a woman will experience several different physiological reactions.

• *Excitement*—vaginal lubrication, a thickening of the vaginal walls and labia, swelling or enlargement of the clitoris

• *Plateau*—expansion of the vagina, coloring of the labia, withdrawal of the clitoris, secretions from Bartholin's gland (preorgasm)

• *Orgasm*—between 5 and 122 contractions occurring approximately every 0.8 seconds, followed by a further 3 to 6 contractions of the sphincter and urethra

• *Resolution*—labia return to normal size and coloration, clitoris returns to normal position, vagina size decreases

It is possible for women to go immediately from the orgasmic stage back to the plateau stage, and from there they can continue love-making and have further orgasms.

Physical reactions in the rest of the body include erect nipples, facial flushing, sweating, hyperventilation, rapid heartbeat, and muscular contractions—and of course there can be an indescribably intense emotional response in addition to the physical reactions.

RIGHT *When women orgasm they experience a series of intense physical sensations.*

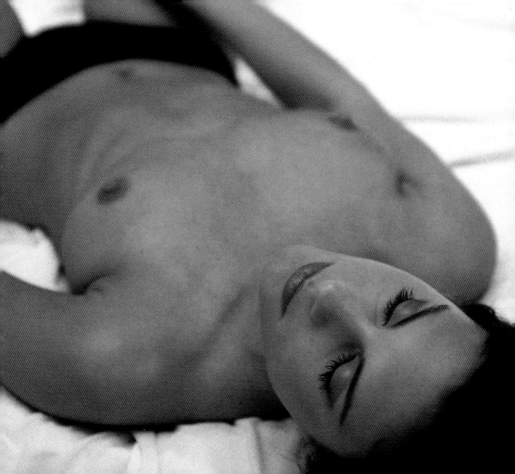

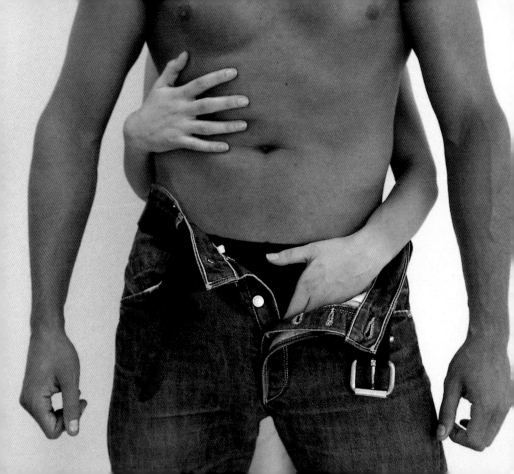

All About the Male Orgasm

Although male orgasm is normally associated with ejaculation, there's a good deal more to it than that, and once you understand the pre-ejaculation phases, you will see how it is possible for men as well as women to have multiple orgasms—a technique that is explained later in the book. In fact, men almost have the advantage, since the stages of their sexual arousal are easily visible—erection of the penis is only the first sign of excitement.

FOR MEN, as for women, there are four phases of orgasm. They are:
• *Excitement*—penile erection, thickening, flattening, and elevation of the scrotal sac, partial testicular elevation, and an increase in size of the penis
• *Plateau*—increase in penile cirumference, testicular swelling, change in hue of penis head to deep purple, secretion from Cowper's gland (preorgasm)
• *Orgasm*—ejaculation accompanied by contractions of vas deferens, seminal vesicles,

LEFT *Erection of the penis is only one sign of male arousal—the whole body becomes excited.*

prostate, and ejaculatory duct; contractions of penile urethra at 0.8 seconds for 3 to 4 contractions; followed by 2 to 4 anal sphincter contractions
• *Resolution*—loss of penile erection

Once ejaculation has taken place, a man cannot immediately have further orgasms.

Again, a man will experience physical reactions throughout his entire body, including erect nipples, facial flushing, hypertension, rapid heartbeat, loss of feeling and numbness, and sweating. As with women, a man's emotional response can be intense and indescribable.

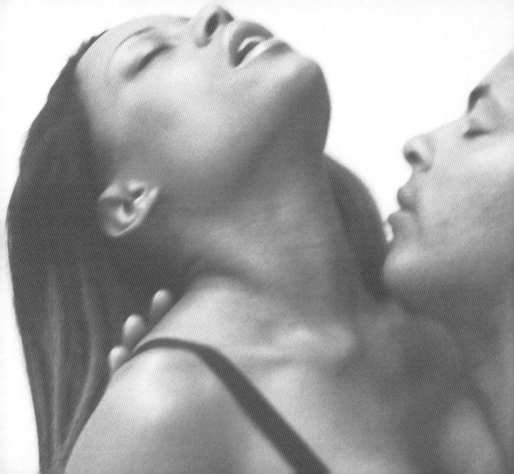

Arousal and Excitement

It has always been assumed or understood that men become sexually aroused more easily than women, that they reach orgasm more quickly, and that they are ready to have sex again sooner. Modern research has shown, however, that this is far from the truth. Some men may indeed become aroused more easily, but some women are just as capable of instant excitement and easy orgasm as their partners.

When it comes to sex, there are simply no rules. Don't make assumptions based on what you think you know—discuss your partner's needs as well as your own. Also, be sensitive to the fact that your individual needs will vary as you go through the cycles of sexuality that are often linked to your mood and what is happening in your life.

Setting the Scene

Sometimes the desire for sexual gratification is sudden, urgent, and spontaneous, but more often we need—or simply desire—to go through the seductive process of flirtation and arousal first. Making love is an act of respect and intimacy, and creating the right atmosphere will demonstrate a thoughtful and considerate approach that may greatly enhance the outcome.

TAKE A LITTLE time and trouble setting the scene for lovemaking—crisp, clean bed linens, soft, warm candlelight, your favorite music, and the scent of fresh flowers will all add to the romantic atmosphere. Take a shower together—this will not only make you feel and smell good, but you can start your mutual seduction as you lather each other. Then wrap yourselves up in fluffy towels, and perhaps share a massage using a sensual aromatherapy oil. A long, gradual increase in arousal as you caress each other, first nonsexually and then more intimately, will help you both feel emotionally safe and wanted as well as physically desired.

If you follow these steps, the anticipation will be exquisite. Anticipation is a very important aspect of lovemaking, because it seems that for both men and women, a prolonged arousal stage leads to a more intense orgasm. For men, a long arousal leads to a greater increase in the size of the testicles and in the thickening, flattening, and elevation of the scrotal sac. In women, prolonged excitement leads to the moistening and expansion of the vagina and the elevation of the cervix. For both sexes, feelings of emotional intimacy intensify greatly.

RIGHT *Spend some time creating the right atmosphere for your lovemaking.*

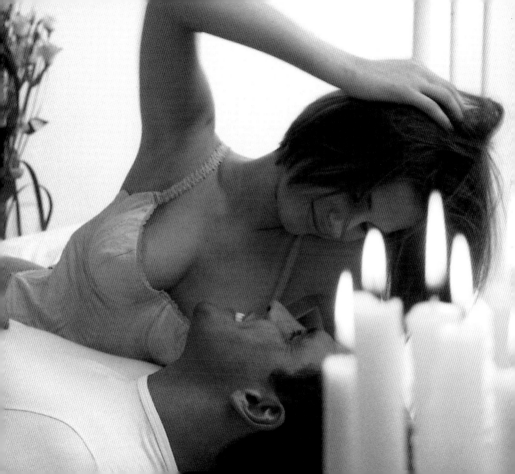

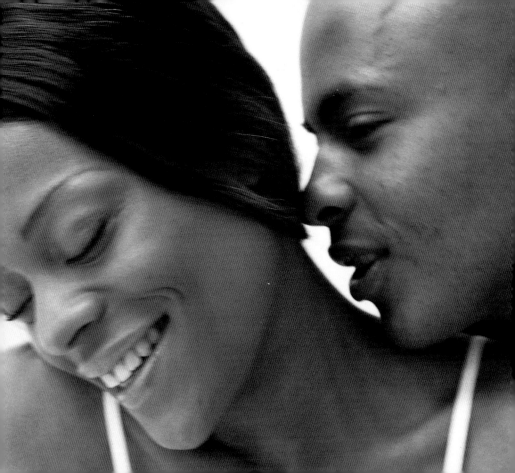

Seduction, Arousal, and Excitement

Understanding the physical process of sexual arousal and orgasm is important because you need to know what is going on if you want to achieve maximum satisfaction from lovemaking. But just knowing which parts of your body go where and how they all work will not necessarily help anything. To achieve truly sensational orgasms, you need to have a good knowledge of what is happening on an emotional level for both your partner and yourself.

IT IS SAID that 90 percent of sex takes place in the mind, so it is here that a deep mutual understanding is needed. It was once thought that men were aroused only by visual stimuli and women only by emotional ones. But recent evidence suggests that, in fact, men and women need similar stimuli—both need to feel wanted, desired, and lusted after. Both need to feel that sex is exciting and sometimes unpredictable. Both partners need to feel that

LEFT *The seduction that occurs before lovemaking determines how exciting it will be. Making your partner feel attractive and desirable through words and actions is vital.*

they are being seduced rather than being taken for granted. Basically, both men and women need to be made to feel that they are sensual and sexy.

If you are to have sensational orgasms as a climax to lovemaking, you need to know that getting there involves reassuring your partner—through words and actions—that you are aware that meeting their emotional needs is a key aspect of satisfying their physical needs. Part of this is knowing what stirs sexual excitement and arousal in your partner—and, perhaps almost as importantly, what does not.

If you and your partner are both really committed to enhancing your orgasms, then you need to explore the aspects of excitement and arousal, and you need to explore them together. This is not something either of you can do in isolation—if you try to achieve this without discussing it together, you will only be going on guesswork and assumptions.

There are no rules or guidelines to be followed—just whatever each of you needs is fine—but it is essential that you feel totally secure and uninhibited with one another and with the relationship, as you need to be able to talk freely about what makes you feel sexually aroused.

You may feel a little shy about this at first, but it's a hurdle you must overcome! Remember to approach this discussion with sensitivity, however. If you have been in the relationship long enough to feel secure with each other, the chances are that you have also been lovers for a while, so it needs to be made clear that the aim of this exercise is not to make your partner feel that he or she has failed to satisfy you sexually up until now—it is to find ways to make a good thing sensational.

Once you have established what arouses each of you, take time to put into practice what you have learned. As you do so, build your confidence by giving feedback—just saying "that feels wonderful" or letting out a little murmur of satisfaction may be enough for you and your partner to let each other know that you are hitting the right spot.

RIGHT *In order to become fully aroused women, and men, need to feel secure and uninhibited. Tell your partner what feels good, and when you are excited, let them know it!*

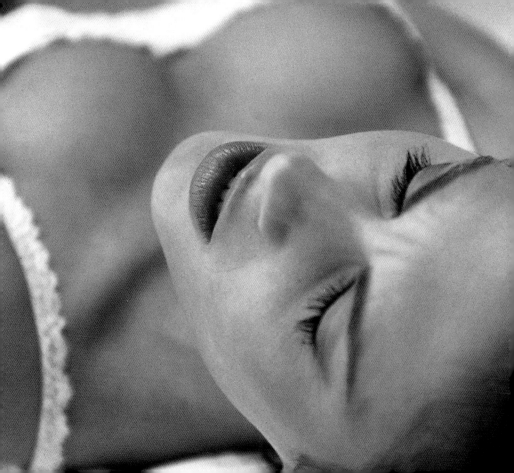

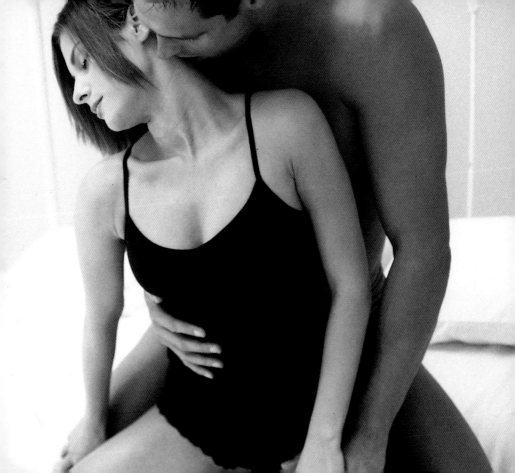

Erogenous Zones

Erogenous zones are those parts of the body that respond with sexual arousal when they are caressed, licked, sucked, teased, tickled, stroked, or kissed. Traditionally, the obvious areas such as the nipples, sexual organs, buttocks, and lips were defined as the erogenous zones, but it is now recognized that this is too limited a definition.

THE SKIN IS FULL of nerves that feel marvelous when touched and stroked. One person may find the backs of the knees sexually sensitive, while another may have the same experience with the nape of the neck or the insides of their thighs.

Are you aware of your partner's erogenous zones? Do you spend time stroking them when you make love? Can you bring your partner to orgasm purely by caressing these areas? Does your partner know where your erogenous zones are and how you like them stimulated?

LEFT *Spend some time with your partner discovering all of your erogenous zones.*

We have already seen that prolonged arousal can lead to sensational orgasms, so it makes sense to use the erogenous zones to enhance that arousal. Using your tongue, lips, and fingers, it is possible to create peaks of such intense sensual pleasure and excitement that your partner will be well on the way to a sensational orgasm before you even touch his or her sexual organs.

Try discovering each other's erogenous zones through massage. Using a massage oil or body lotion, take turns stroking one another's whole body—front and back, arms and legs, hands and feet—erotically but not sexually, and communicate your reactions.

Foreplay

Is foreplay really a part of lovemaking, or is it just a quick appetizer? Is it necessary, and for how long should it go on? What does it involve anyway? Is it just a little preliminary kissing, or do you include a bit of sexual touching as well?

FIRST OF ALL, drop any idea you might have that foreplay and sex are separate activities. Of course, you can have foreplay without sex, although you may find it difficult to concentrate on anything else afterward! You can also have sex without foreplay, but arousal will be incomplete and the act of sex will be simply that—sex, and probably unsatisfactory sex at that, unless you are both in the mood to just go for it.

Foreplay is all about arousal—kissing, erotic caressing, licking, and sucking, with plenty of skin-to-skin contact—so it is absolutely necessary. You can devote as much time and attention as you like to this stage, until your mutual excitement is overwhelming.

At this stage, the desire to move on becomes irresistible. But don't give up on foreplay at this point—maintain contact through fingers, lips, tongues, and hands. Continue to stroke and caress the erogenous nerve endings to keep them stimulated. By doing this, you will ensure that the transition from erotic arousal to sexual touching is smooth and flowing. Excitement will remain at its maximum level throughout your lovemaking, and there will be a corresponding level of sensational orgasm.

RIGHT *Foreplay is essential to sensational lovemaking and the longer it lasts the better. Keep up the kissing, caressing, and licking as you move on to sexual touching.*

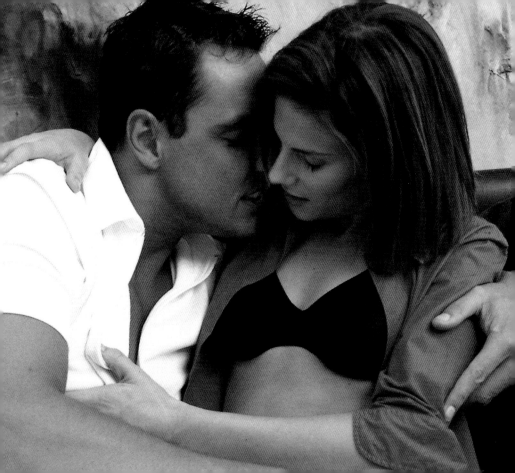

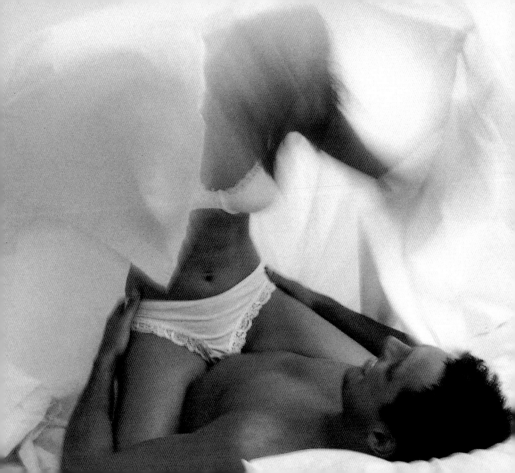

Helping Each Other to Sensational Orgasm

Although it is possible for almost everyone to achieve quite a satisfactory orgasm through masturbation, you need a partner in order to achieve a sensational orgasm. To share the ultimate climax with your partner, you both need to feel safe, relaxed, and desired.

BEFORE EMBARKING on the techniques and exercises on the following pages, it is a good idea to ascertain just how comfortable you feel with each other. You need to be totally familiar not only with your own body and sexual responses, but also with your partner's. Take some time to answer the following questions honestly.

• How comfortable are you being naked with each other?
• Are you both familiar with the other person's sexual organs?
• Do you each know how the other likes to achieve orgasm?

LEFT *Find out how comfortable you and your partner feel with each other's bodies.*

• Can you bring each other to orgasm easily and frequently?
• Is there anything about your own sexuality that embarrasses you?
• Is there anything about your partner's sexuality that embarrasses you?
• Are you both excited at the prospect of enhancing the quality of your orgasms?

Discuss and resolve any issues related to your responses before you go any further. Then discuss what goals you are setting, what you expect to achieve, and how you will monitor your progress—but try not to get too clinical, as the aim is to bring you and your partner emotionally and physically closer together, not to give you a new problem!

Mutual Masturbation

It is not always easy to focus on your partner's orgasm when you are close to climax yourself,
but with mutual masturbation coordination is important. Get the timing right, and you can
both achieve a sensational orgasm—almost, if not always absolutely, simultaneously—far more
easily than by having full-on sex in any position. Mutual masturbation is also ideal if either
of you is tired or unable to take a fully active role for any reason.

BEGIN YOUR mutual masturbation by warming up with the foreplay exercises on page 30. Continue until you are both fully aroused. Once you feel ready, it is usually easiest if the woman lies on her back and the man kneals at her side. This position gives her good access to his penis, and she can play with his testicles. At the same time, he can lean over her to suck and lick her breasts and caress her clitoris. He can also insert the fingers of his other hand into her vagina to stimulate deep inside her. The woman can masturbate the man hard and fast in this position without tiring.

If you want to climax together, it is helpful if you can learn to recognize each other's signals for approaching orgasm. These might include faster breathing, writhing, gasping, and so on. If one of you is approaching orgasm faster than the other, you can slow down the stimulation or ease up for a moment. Obviously it is not absolutely essential to achieve orgasm at the same time, but it can be thrilling if you do.

RIGHT *Experiment with your partner to find the easiest and most comfortable positions for mutual masturbation. With practice you will be able to achieve orgasm together.*

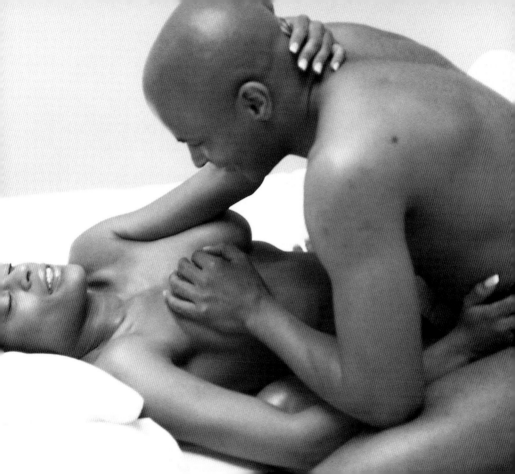

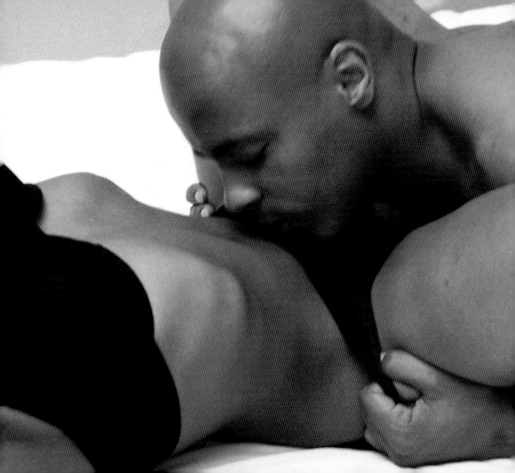

Oral Sex

*If you feel really comfortable with each other, oral sex is a fantastic way to enhance your
orgasms. Oral sex is all about giving pleasure to your partner. Initially, until you are ready, you
should not focus on achieving an orgasm—if you are concentrating only on the climax, you will
miss out on the pleasure of getting there. Remember, as always, that maintaining
communication between you is important.*

SPEND SOME TIME practicing oral sex,
taking it in turns, but without aiming
for an orgasm. The man should use his
tongue to explore the woman's sexual organs,
discovering how she responds as he licks and
sucks each area, and inserting his fingers into
her vagina to explore and stimulate there at
the same time. He should run his tongue up
and down either side of the clitoris, and she
should communicate how this feels. She

LEFT *A man should spend some time
getting to know a woman's sexual organs
using his tongue and fingers at the same
time, and watching her responses.*

should express how it feels when he only licks
her clitoris.

The woman should spend time sucking
her partner's penis, again without trying to
make him climax. She should try varying the
intensity and speed of the suck, and how far
up or down the shaft her tongue goes. She
can also suck his testicles, run her finger up
and down his perineum, and insert a finger
into his rectum.

Try as many techniques as you like until
you are each totally familiar with the other's
responses. Now you can help each other
achieve a sensational orgasm more easily.

Libido and Lovemaking

Inevitably there will be times when you or your partner do not feel like making love. You may be tired, recovering from childbirth, feeling the effects of work stress, convalescing after illness— or you may just not be in the mood. If you put pressure on your partner to have sex at these times, you could destroy the trust you have built up between you.

IF YOUR partner cannot respect your wishes and won't back off when you don't feel like having sex, then you will not be able to relax enough to enjoy great orgasms—part of you will always hang back from total commitment. You may also begin to feel that your relationship is not built on the solid foundation you once believed it to be.

Individuals go through cycles of sexual desire and apathy, and relationships also go through these cycles. A new relationship is nearly always marked by overwhelming desire for each other, which later settles into a comfortable security that might not be as exciting as it was at the beginning. Yet the relationship that develops will hopefully prove to be lasting and satisfying.

If either of you is experiencing a loss of libido, then you must talk about how you feel and how you have arrived at this point. You may think about seeking professional help if the problem is acute or has been an issue for a long time. If one of you simply has a lower libido than the other, however, this is fine and is perfectly natural—just work on having really great sex when the time is right.

RIGHT *If you are experiencing a loss of libido, for whatever reason, it is best to talk to your partner about it before the problems become more serious and harder to deal with.*

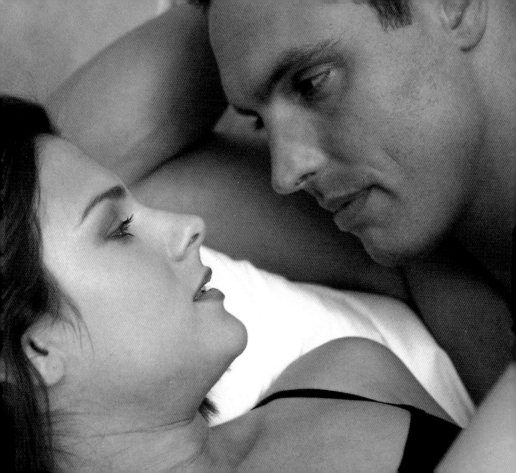

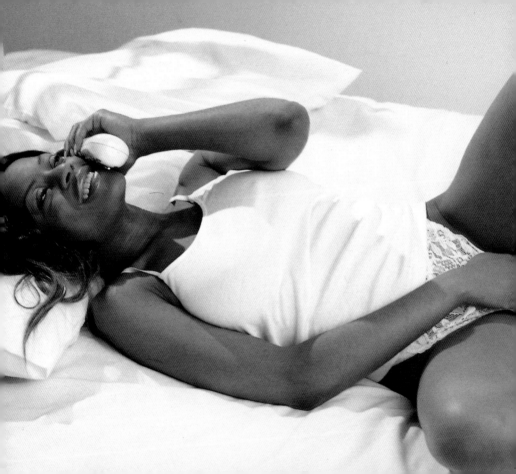

Eroticism and Fantasies

If you want to enhance your orgasms, you need to think about eroticism and fantasy, as these have an important role in love play. Being erotic is all about generating excitement—building up the tension and sexual heat between the two of you so that when you arrive at orgasm it is that much more intense. If you approach sex in a formal way, it will likely be less than satisfactory.

IT IS NORMAL and natural to have fantasies—to dream about having sex with strangers or famous people, or about making love in unusual places or in unusual ways. It is normal and natural to want your lovemaking to be exciting, spontaneous, lustful, and hot. To achieve this, you have to make an effort. You have to talk dirty sometimes—phone your partner with outrageous suggestions or send a letter or e-mail outlining exactly what you would like to do or try the next

LEFT *To make lovemaking more intense, generate excitement and build up sexual tension by talking to your partner about your fantasies beforehand.*

time you make love. Discuss your fantasies together and then help each other live them out. As long as you are secure in your relationship, you shouldn't have a problem with any of this.

Being sexy isn't about taking your clothes off—it's about the way you take them off. It's about what you were wearing in the first place. You need to dress provocatively for your lover if you want to thrill, tease, and please. Talk to your partner about what he or she would like you to wear before making love. As with most things, the more effort you put in and the longer the time you take, the greater the reward.

Sensational Orgasms for Women

This section is for women to work on—either alone or with their partner—so that they feel completely at ease with their sexuality. If you wish to enhance your own and your partner's orgasms, it is essential that you know your way around your sexual organs, so the first section looks at masturbation and self-exploration. These exercises will also help you to achieve sensational orgasms with your partner because, if you are able to bring yourself to orgasm easily and frequently, you can enjoy showing your partner what turns you on.

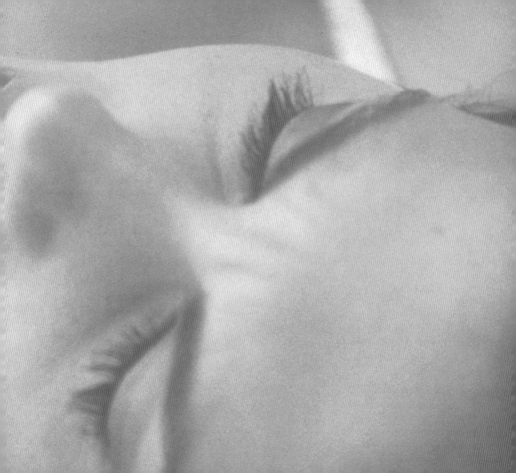

Self-Exploration

For you to have truly sensational orgasms, you need a good knowledge of your own body. Self-exploration and self-loving make perfect sense if you want to achieve mind-blowing orgasms with your partner, so learn to make love to yourself as you would like him to make love to you.

IF YOU HAVE no idea what your sexual parts look like, lie on the bed with your legs apart and place a mirror where you can easily see your genitalia. Explore gently, pulling open the labia and stroking the clitoral hood, so you can see what physical changes occur when you become aroused—see page 16 for more about these changes.

Next, set aside plenty of private time and create the sort of sensual, romantic atmosphere you would like to share with your partner. Stroke your body—erotically at first, noting your body's responses as you touch different areas, then more sexually as you become aroused. Start to stimulate yourself, but take your time—this is a voyage of discovery, not a race. Continue to observe your reactions to the different ways you touch yourself, especially as you reach climax.

Now you need to communicate your findings to your partner. If you feel very comfortable with him, you can carry out this exercise in masturbation in front of him, allowing him to watch so that he knows exactly where and how you would like to be touched. Alternatively, guide him through your discoveries the next time you are making love together.

RIGHT *Take some time to slowly and gently explore your sexual organs, finding out what excites you and the physical changes that occur.*

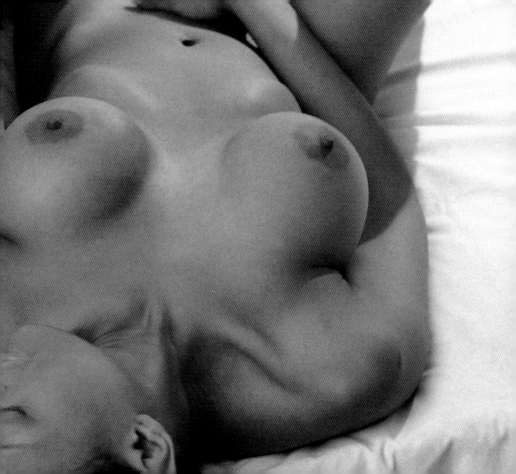

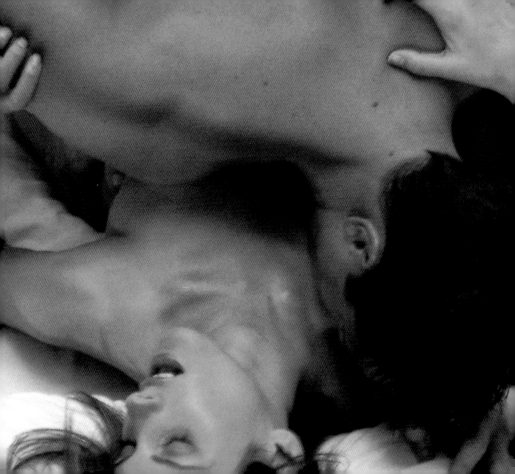

Different Kinds of Orgasm

*For many years it was believed that a woman either didn't have orgasms or, if she did,
it was because her partner thrust hard enough into her during intercourse to bring her to
vaginal orgasm. Now, however, it is recognized that women can have three, if not four,
different types of orgasm.*

VAGINAL ORGASM

Many women find it quite hard to achieve
vaginal orgasm, but it should be not only
possible but also very easy if the vaginal walls
are massaged properly. Some women respond
to long, slow movements, while others need
hard thrusts or perhaps require a combination
of both. Spend some time finding out what
feels best to you, and then communicate with
your partner so he knows exactly how to
bring you to orgasm.

LEFT *Women can have several kinds of
orgasm. With good communication and
practice, a man can learn to bring his
partner to climax in all the different ways.*

CLITORAL ORGASM

The clitoris is extremely sensitive. Caressing
it with care and expertise leads easily to
orgasm. A man can use his tongue, lips, and
fingers on and around the clitoris to bring his
partner to orgasm, but while most women
can achieve a good clitoral orgasm on their
own, they often find it harder if their partner
is trying to bring them to orgasm this way. It
may be best to show your partner what sort
of movement and pressure you like.

G-SPOT ORGASM

The G-spot is located on the underside of
the clitoris, inside the vagina—it is a rougher

area of tissue that can be felt on the upper part of the vagina, about two inches inside. Again, this is a fairly sensitive area and it is best to stimulate either side of it. The man should insert two fingers into the vagina, positioned at 11:00 and 1:00 o'clock, and stroke upward. As his partner starts to climax, he can pull quite hard upward with his fingers to intensify her orgasm, at the same time pushing down hard on her pubic bone with his other hand.

ANAL ORGASM

The anus contains more nerve endings than most parts of the body and is extremely sensitive. However, not all women like the idea of anal sex play, although those who do practice it frequently report intense orgasms.

COMBINATIONS

A woman's orgasm can be greatly intensified if more than one area is stimulated. For example, if you find it exciting to have full

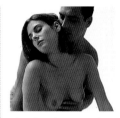

intercourse but you are unable to achieve vaginal orgasm, you can still have an orgasm if your clitoris is stimulated at the same time, either by you or your partner. You may also like your partner to stimulate the anal opening while you are having intercourse.

A man can give his partner a combination orgasm through masturbation, although it may sound like he needs three hands to do so! However, it can be achieved with just one hand. He can use his index finger and his forefinger to stimulate the woman's vagina by massaging the G-spot, his thumb to caress the clitoris, and his little finger to enter the anus. His free hand can then be used to stroke and caress his partner's breasts.

RIGHT *Experiment with stimulating several areas to produce an intense orgasm.*

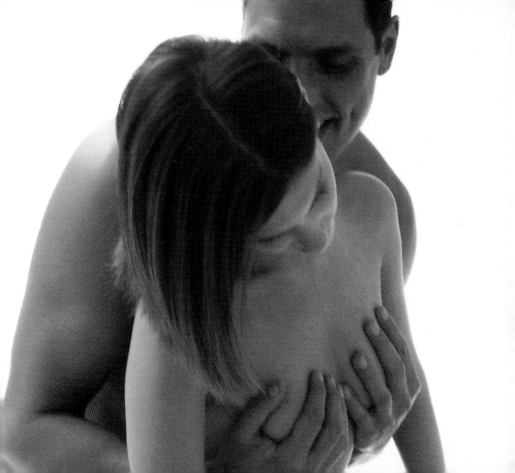

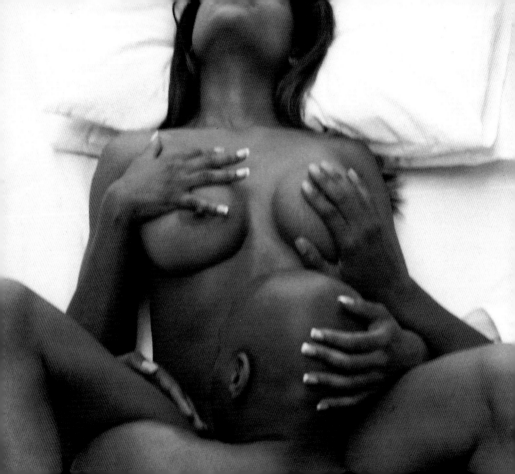

Suck, Don't Blow

The clitoris is made up of erectile tissue—it stands up and out when a woman is sexually excited. Your partner can bring you to a truly sensational orgasm through oral sex if he uses some of the same techniques that you use on him—sucking as well as licking. This technique needs a certain finesse, as the clitoris is sensitive and will withdraw if the friction is too extreme.

YOUR PARTNER SHOULD take the clitoris into his mouth and suck on it with his lips, sliding his tongue gently over the very tip of the clitoris as he does so. The sucking should be firm but very gentle, and the woman should communicate her reactions clearly, as some women can take quite extreme sucking while others find the technique too pleasurable for words and simply can't stand the exquisite sensations it produces. If this is the case and the pleasure is

LEFT *Oral stimulation can produce a mind-blowing clitoral orgasm. The man should alternate between sucking and licking depending on the woman's responses.*

simply overwhelming, suggest to your partner that he alternates between licking and sucking, switching from licking to sucking without warning, then going back to licking when the sucking sensation becomes too intense for you to stand.

Your partner can also roll the clitoris around his tongue instead of sucking or licking by drawing the clitoris into his mouth as if he were sucking the juice from an orange, or he can gently pull the clitoris up between his tongue and top teeth. These techniques can be extremely pleasurable, but your partner should be very careful not to bite or blow.

Multiple Orgasms

It is said that women can have multiple orgasms much more easily than men can, and although this may be true, there are many women who have yet to experience multiple orgasms. There may also be many women who are experiencing prolonged single orgasms, which other women would describe as multiple orgasms.

IF AN ORGASM lasts quite a few minutes and comes in waves with peaks and troughs, should this be considered one orgasm or multiple orgasms? It all depends on how you determine "multiple." Technically, a multiple orgasm is a series of separate orgasms with a definite resolution stage between each one—see page 16. That being the case, a single orgasm that comes in waves and lasts a long time is still technically only one.

So if you have not experienced multiple orgasms, how do you do so? It's all in the timing. If your partner begins arousal through foreplay too long after the resolution stage of your orgasm, your body will have "closed down" and feel tired, and it will be harder to arouse you again and bring you back to an orgasmic state.

However, if your partner begins foreplay again within a very short space of time, you will be much more responsive and will come back to an orgasmic state much more quickly, and possibly with increasing intensity because the sexual organs are in a state of heightened sensitivity. If you delay, the fuse grows cold. Begin again quickly, though, and the heat is retained. It really is as simple as that.

RIGHT *It is easy to bring a woman to multiple orgasms. Simply begin foreplay again shortly after she climaxes.*

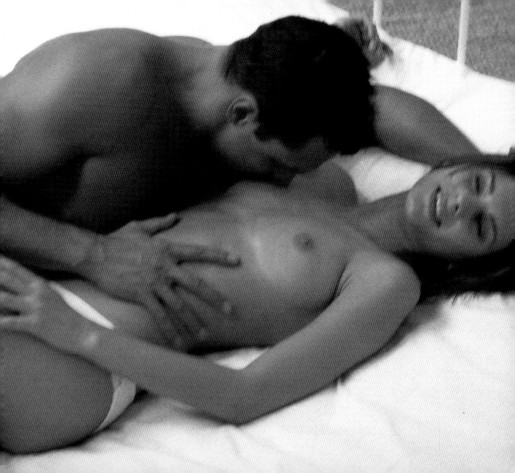

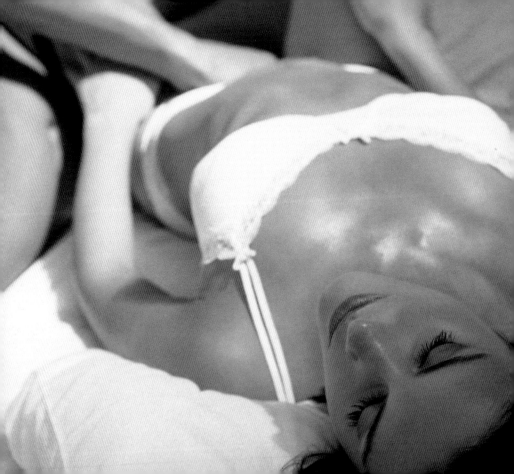

Feeling the Quality

We have already looked at women's three—or four—orgasmic zones, so now it's time to explore how your partner can bring some or all of them into play at the same time in order to help you achieve a truly sensational orgasm. To start, your partner needs to imagine that your sexual organs are a piece of fine and expensive cloth, and that he is going to feel the quality.

To DO THIS, he would take the cloth between his thumb and his index and middle fingers, and rub it gently with his thumb. He can use the same technique to stimulate you by inserting his index and

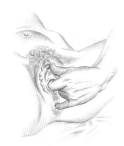

RIGHT *The thumb stimulates the clitoris, two fingers massage the G-spot, and the little finger is inserted into the woman's anus.*

LEFT *Stimulating all of the erogenous zones at the same time brings a sensational orgasm.*

middle fingers into your vagina and feeling for the G-spot, and then by using his thumb to massage your clitoris.

He should do this quite gently to begin with, and should gradually increase the tempo, making small, circular movements around and across the clitoris. The two fingers inside should be positioned at 11:00 and 1:00 o'clock so they can move up and down on either side of your G-spot. He can pull upward quite hard as you reach your climax, and you should enjoy a sensational orgasm in both places simultaneously. He can also insert the little finger of the same hand into your rectum if you enjoy this type of stimulation.

Sensational Orgasms for Men

This section is for men to work on—either alone or with their partner—so that they feel completely at ease with their sexuality. If you wish to enhance your own orgasms, as well as your partner's, it is essential that you know your way around your sexual organs. It will also help you to achieve sensational orgasms with your partner if you are able to bring yourself to orgasm easily and frequently. Once you know what excites you, you can teach your partner. They can then bring in some of the different skills covered in this section—from manual stimulation to great oral sex techniques.

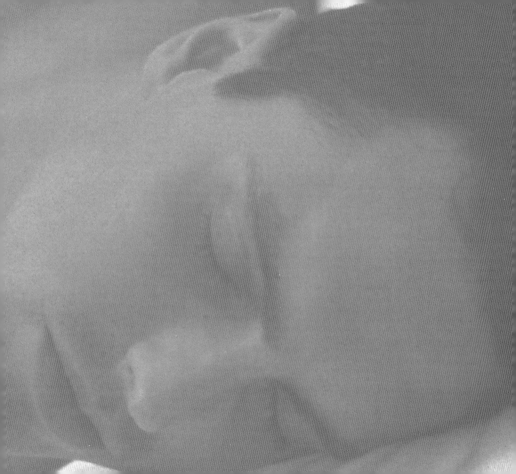

Delaying and Stopping Male Orgasm

Before men can enhance their orgasms, they have to learn to control them. This means being able to delay an orgasm on demand. If you and your partner want to practice simultaneous orgasms, you need to be able to stop your orgasm if necessary and "wait" for your partner.

EARLIER, WE LOOKED at the four phases of orgasm—excitement, plateau, orgasm, and resolution. The easiest point at which to delay or stop an orgasm is during the plateau stage. Since it takes a lot more control to stop an orgasm as it happens, it is better to recognize the "warning" signs of orgasm and to stop any further stimulation before it is too late.

You should practice by masturbating—with or without your partner—and when you feel the ejaculate starting to rise, stop stroking or rubbing your penis until the feeling subsides. Then start again, and again stop when you feel the ejaculate starting to rise. By careful monitoring, it is possible to

bring yourself right up to the point of orgasm, and then stop.

Other techniques that stop orgasm include squeezing the head of the penis or clutching hard at the scrotum, but you may not wish to apply pressure to your sensitive parts.

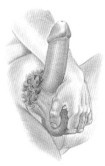

RIGHT *Clutching at the scrotum delays orgasm. Pinching the skin between the scrotum and anus will also do this.*

OPPOSITE PAGE *Squeezing the head of the penis is one way to stop a man from reaching orgasm.*

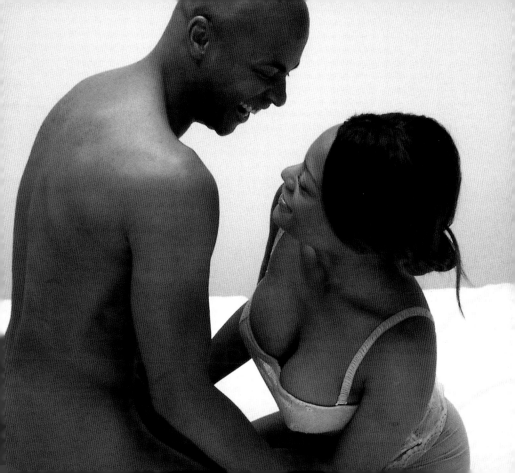

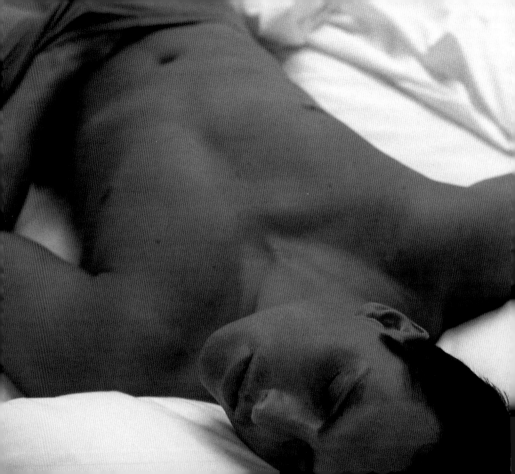

Intensifying the Male Orgasm

One of the ways in which you can help to create a sensational orgasm is by strengthening the action of a muscle located roughly under the prostate gland, called the pubococcygeus, or PC muscle. As you start to orgasm, the PC muscle will pulse or throb, causing the ejaculate to be pumped up from the prostate gland—where it is mixed with the semen—and then out through the penis.

IF YOU STOP masturbating—or thrusting inside your partner if you are having intercourse—exactly at the moment of orgasm, you will be able to feel the PC muscle contract violently inside you. The stronger this muscle is, the more intense your orgasm will be.

If you need help locating your PC muscle, the next time you urinate, try to stop the flow before you are finished. When you do

LEFT *Practice stopping masturbation just at the moment of orgasm so that you can feel the PC muscle contract inside you. Use this technique to intensify your orgasms.*

this, the muscle you feel contracting is the PC muscle. Once you have found it, it is easy to start strengthening the muscle by alternately contracting and relaxing it—you can do this while sitting down or relaxing in bed. Spend a few minutes each day practicing, and the muscle will soon become much stronger. Then, when you are at the point of orgasm— just when you feel the first spurt start—you can contract the muscle and feel the intensity of your orgasm leap.

With practice, it should be possible for you to achieve orgasm simply by repeatedly squeezing this muscle.

Dealing with Overexcitement

Premature ejaculation—to give it its clinical title—is when a man ejaculates too easily.
It most often happens, completely involuntarily, just as he puts his penis into his partner's
vagina. If premature ejaculation is seen as a problem, especially by the woman, it tends
to get worse rather than better.

IT IS WORTH bearing in mind that some men suffer from the opposite of premature ejaculation—retarded ejaculation—a condition in which a man has no difficulty getting and maintaining an erection, but finds it hard to ejaculate. This condition can cause frustration and stress within a relationship.

Premature ejaculation can be overcome by decreasing the sensitivity of the penis. The way to do this is to work on increasing the level of stimulation a man can endure before he ejaculates. A couple can practice by using any of the various masturbation techniques in this book, but the one for delaying or stopping orgasms is particularly valuable.

Another method, which is probably much better, is simply to allow the man to ejaculate when it happens naturally, without making an issue of it, and then to immediately stimulate the penis so that he doesn't lose his erection. The couple can then carry on making love and the man need not feel any regret, guilt, or loss of self-esteem. His second ejaculation may not be as intense, but it will certainly be harder to achieve, allowing him to make love for much longer. It is extremely unlikely that he will experience a series of premature ejaculations.

RIGHT *Lovemaking can continue if a man*
is stimulated again right after orgasm.

62

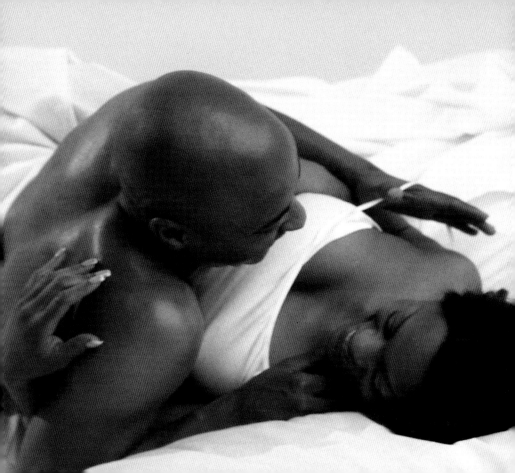

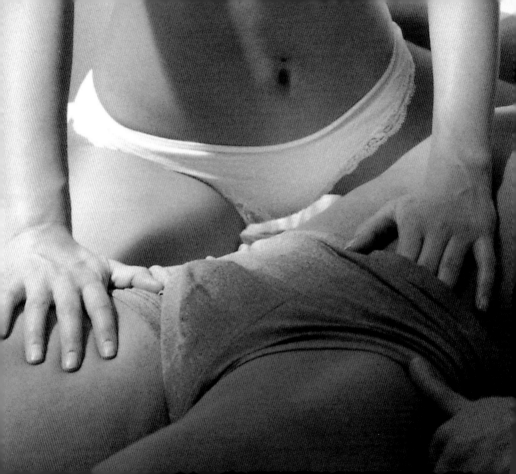

Creative Use of the Hands

Here are some methods that your partner can use to give you a truly sensational orgasm by masturbating you. Most men need fast hand action to achieve orgasm, but with clever and creative use of her hands, your partner can increase your pleasure range without tiring herself.

THE TWO-HANDED PUMP

With one hand tightly wrapped around the base of your penis and the other around the top, your partner brings her hands together in a pumping action. As her hands meet in the middle of your penis, the slamming effect will produce considerable pressure and intense stimulation, leading to a sensational orgasm.

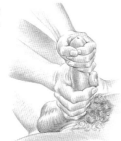

RIGHT *The hands should be positioned in this way for the two-handed pump and the two-handed twist.*

LEFT *Using creative methods, a woman can give her partner a great orgasm without exhausting herself.*

THE TWO-HANDED TWIST

Your partner places her hands in the same position as for the two-handed pump, but twists them in opposite directions. It may take you longer to reach orgasm this way, but it should still be sensational.

THE BALL STRETCH

Your partner wraps one hand around the base of your penis and pulls down toward your testicles quite hard. The other fist masturbates you. If she keeps up the pressure on the downward pull, your climax will be explosive.

Sensational Oral Orgasm

The best position for you to be in if you want to be given a sensational oral orgasm is sitting with your legs across your partner's thighs. You can then lie back or sit upright, and your partner will have full access to your penis and testicles. This is important because she will need to exert lots of firm pressure in order for you to get all the stimulation you need to orgasm in this position.

S HE SHOULD START by using her saliva to moisten your penis all over. She can do this very gently at first with her lips and tongue, and she can then use her tongue to circle the head of the penis as she starts to stroke it. After a few downward strokes she can take the head of the penis into her mouth and suck quite hard. As her hand travels downward, she should follow with her mouth, and as her mouth travels upward again, she should follow once again with her hand. The upward suck and stroke should be lighter than the downward one, which should be extremely firm.

Your partner can pause occasionally to lick the head of the penis, paying special attention to the underside, and tugging gently on your testicles. As you start to orgasm, it will be sensational if your partner coordinates your ejaculation with her last strong downward pull and suck, making sure she has as much of your penis in her mouth as possible. The penis will shrink slightly as you ejaculate, so a firm grip and a deep suck are extremely important.

RIGHT *Find a comfortable position that gives your partner good access to your penis and testicles.*

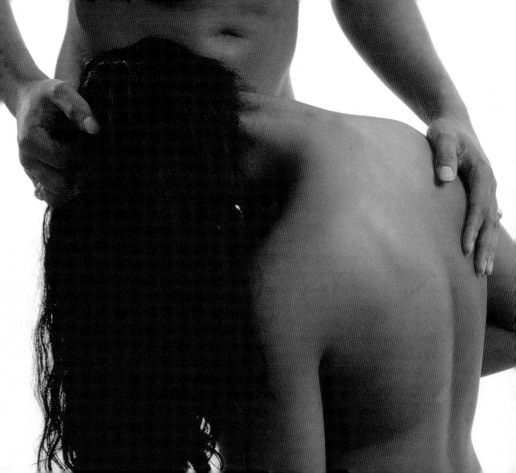

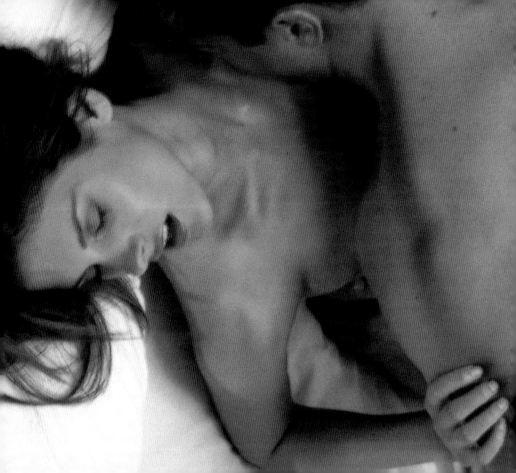

Multiple Orgasms for Men

If women can have multiple orgasms, why can't men? Well, they can. It takes a little more practice as well as a movement away from being too focused on the ejaculation as the prime goal of the orgasm. Men can orgasm without having to ejaculate. Once they accept this, they are ready to move toward becoming multiorgasmic.

WE LOOKED EARLIER at how you can use the PC muscle to strengthen and intensify the male orgasm. Well, this same muscle can be used to encourage multiple orgasms in men. You can do the following exercise with your partner or alone.

Start by stroking the penis until it is erect. When you feel yourself entering the final stages of excitement and the semen is starting to rise, stop all movement. You will need to breathe deeply as you tightly clench the PC muscle, but if you have strengthened the

LEFT *With practice, men can learn to orgasm without having to ejaculate, enabling them to have multiple orgasms.*

muscle by exercising it vigorously, you should be able to stop the ejaculation. Keep in mind that you won't actually stop the orgasm, and you will still feel the same sensations you have with an ejaculatory orgasm. Once the need to ejaculate has passed, though, you can start stroking again. The penis will not subside as it would after ejaculation takes place.

You can again come to a peak just prior to ejaculation, stop and clench, breathe deeply, and stop the ejaculation while still having the orgasm. There is technically no limit to the number of times you can do this, but you should always try to finish with an ejaculatory orgasm.

Simultaneous Orgasms

This section is about achieving orgasms together, which, although not essential, does seem to be a natural goal for many couples. There is something very loving about having simultaneous orgasms. However, it is important you are able to enjoy your own orgams and are not too focused on making sure your partner is also climaxing. Once you have practiced ways of achieving simultaneous orgasm, whether through masturbation or full intercourse, you can start to enhance your shared orgasms to a sensational level.

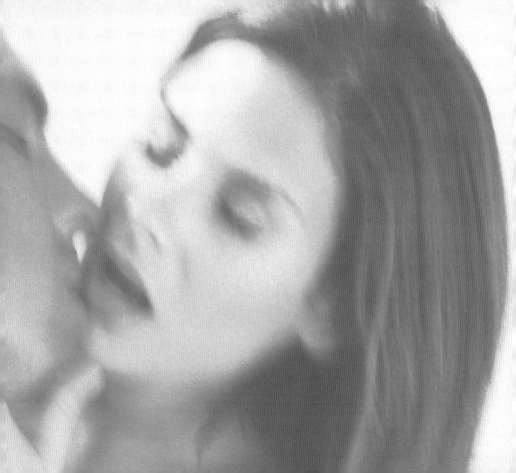

Simultaneous Orgasm Through Masturbation

*One of the easiest ways to enjoy a simultaneous orgasm is by masturbation. This way
you can time and pace your orgasms to coincide. Good communication is essential here,
as you each need to know what is happening to your partner and either be able to wait
or ask your partner to wait, if necessary.*

START OFF LYING side by side, and spend plenty of time caressing each other until you are both aroused—the woman should be feeling moist and the man's penis should be fully erect. When you are ready, each of you should use one hand to start masturbating yourself, while your other hand continues to caress your partner. For example, the man can use his fingers to caress the outer lips of his partner's vagina, while the woman can caress her partner's scrotum and perineum. As you touch each other, talk about how excited you are feeling, especially when you are nearing your climax. You should be able to time it so that you orgasm at the same time.

You can also try this masturbation exercise lying feet to head so that you can touch each other from a different angle. For example, the man can insert his fingers into his partner's vagina when he is lying in this position. This kind of visual stimulation can also prove to be very exciting.

Once you have learned how to achieve simultaneous orgasm by masturbating yourselves, you can move on to masturbating one another.

RIGHT *As you each touch yourselves and each other, talk about how excited you are feeling so that you can attempt to achieve a simultaneous orgasm.*

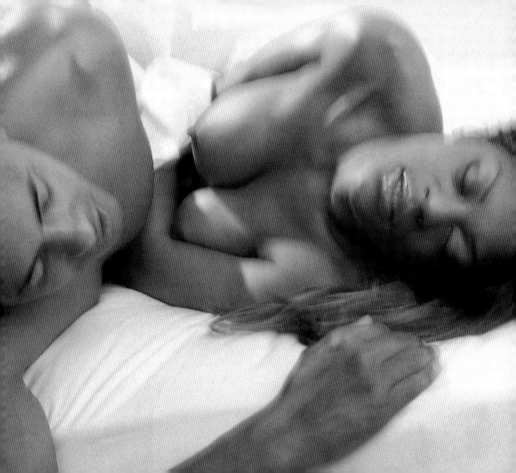

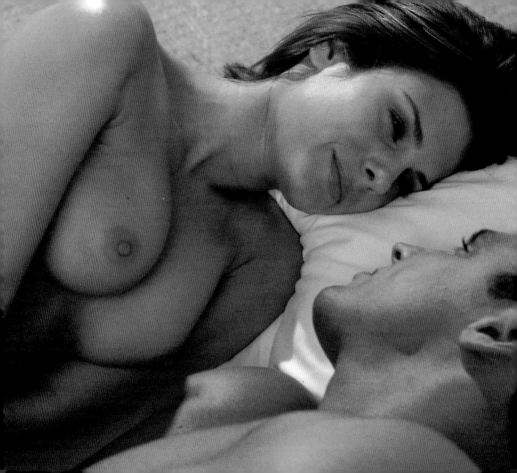

Mutual Masturbation

Once you are used to gauging the progress of your own orgasms while both masturbating and caressing yourselves, it is not difficult to continue this exercise by masturbating each other. Again, you should lie side by side to start off and caress each other until you are both excited enough to begin.

THE MAN CAN help his partner while she masturbates him by caressing his scrotum and perineum while she touches his penis. The woman can caress her outer vaginal lips while her partner strokes and rubs her clitoris. Again, it is essential that good communication is kept up so that you can alter the timing and tempo of your technique. At certain stages one of you may need to slow down so that neither of you achieves orgasm before the other.

LEFT *Once you have practiced this technique you will be able to experience enjoyable lovemaking even if one partner is tired or experiencing low libido.*

There will be times when it doesn't work, and one of you comes first, but that doesn't matter. This exercise should be very enjoyable in addition to being a learning exercise. Gradually it will become easier to time it so that you achieve orgasm at the same time— in this case, practice makes perfect.

This exercise and the previous one are ideal when you don't want to or cannot have a full bout of lovemaking. It is also a useful alternative when one partner is experiencing low libido since it doesn't require too much in the way of preparation or foreplay, but the technique does ultimately bring orgasmic relief in a state of togetherness.

Masturbation and Oral Sex

Another technique to add to your lovemaking skills is masturbating while performing oral sex. There are several variations on this theme, and you can practice them all in turn until you know each other's orgasmic routines. Once you know the signs and signals, you will be able to time it so that simultaneous orgasms become easy.

To START WITH, the woman can suck her partner's penis and rub it with one hand while she masturbates herself with the other. He can use his free hands to stroke her breasts and face. She can then time her own orgasm to coincide with her partner ejaculating into her mouth.

You can then change positions so that the man can lick and suck his partner's clitoris while masturbating himself. If she lies back and he kneels between her legs, the man has good access to his penis while his partner can pull up hard on her pubic region to give him good access to her clitoris and vagina. In this position, communication is difficult for the man, so his partner will have to be clear about her level of excitement and how near she is to orgasm—moans and groans might be misinterpreted. The man will find it fun, helpful, and exciting if his partner "talks dirty" to him about how she's feeling.

If you like a challenge you can now try the classic position known as "69," where you each have access to stimulate one another orally. Simultaneous orgasm in this position is probably the hardest of all to achieve. The penis is designed to point upward, and in this position it is being forced downward into the

RIGHT *In this position the woman enjoys oral sex while the man masturbates himself.*

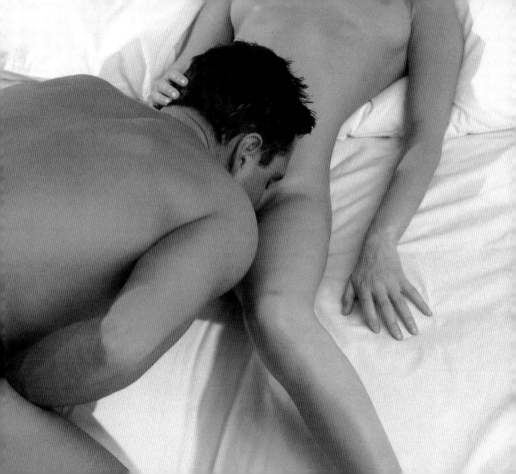

woman's mouth. Many men and women find it difficult to orgasm in this position, but it is worth persevering, as it is exciting and a lot of fun to try, even if simultaneous orgasm doesn't happen.

In this position, the woman can masturbate her clitoris while her partner pushes his tongue deep inside her, and the man can masturbate himself as his penis is taken into her mouth. This all sounds a little athletic, but it just requires practice.

These techniques rely on you knowing your own and your partner's sexual preferences. This is one of the reasons that this book is designed for loving couples in stable relationships—you simply wouldn't do some of these things on a first date. But lovemaking is at its best when you are both relaxed enough to try new things and have new experiences and are prepared to practice until you achieve what you want.

RIGHT *The classic "69" oral-sex position requires a little practice to get it right.*

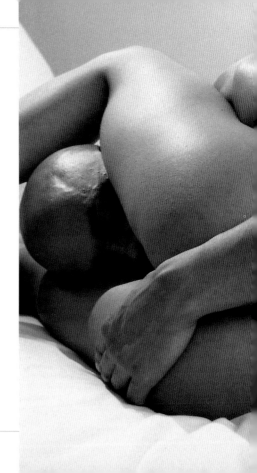

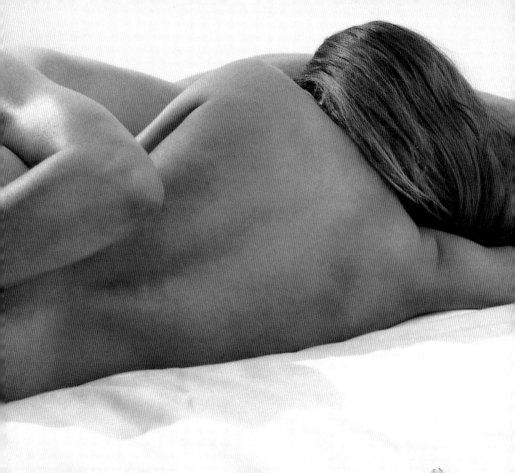

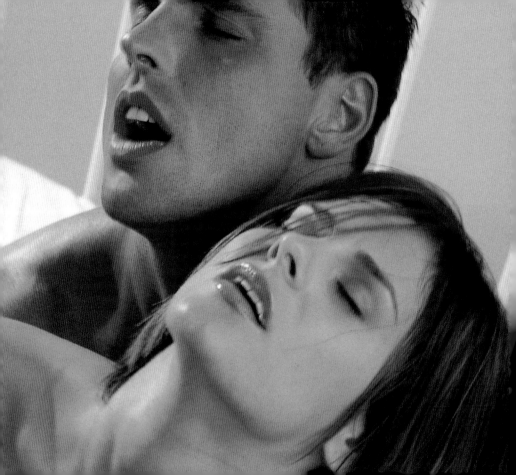

The Reciprocal Orgasm

Sometimes it's great to have simultaneous orgasms, but it is also important to be allowed to concentrate on your own orgasm without having to do anything else at the same time. Once one of you has come, and recovered, you can then change things around so that the other person can come too.

SOMETIMES it's great to be given an orgasm by your partner and not to have to reciprocate afterward. There is perhaps no greater gift in a relationship than to give your partner a sensational orgasm and expect nothing in return except the pleasure of watching your lover fall asleep in a glow of sexual satisfaction.

This is another good alternative to a full bout of lovemaking if one of you is experiencing low libido.

LEFT *The ability to give selflessly is vital in all good relationships. If you are able to give your partner an orgasm without expecting one in return, you are truly a great lover.*

If you want to be a great lover, why not aim to be the best lover your partner could ever want? It's easy to do. Ask your partner what he or she wants—what he or she would like you to do, and how he or she would like their orgasm to happen.

To be the very best, all it takes is the ability to listen and to deliver what is required. If this can be done in a selfless way, then really good sex is easy. So, the next session covers reciprocal orgasms. If you are giving your partner an orgasm first, allow him or her time to recover before receiving yours. Remember, you are offering each other an honor, a favor, and a gift that should be savored, not rushed.

Simultaneous Orgasm Through Intercourse

Once you know each other's orgasmic phases really well, you might like to move on to having simultaneous orgasms while you are having intercourse. This is harder to achieve, but it can be done if you use the masturbation techniques described earlier in this book.

THOSE SCENARIOS you see in the movies, where a man thrusts his penis into his lover's vagina and miraculously brings both partners to climax at the same time, are totally unrealistic. This kind of thing does not usually happen except by accident, and even then it is very rare. Some couples can share an entire lifetime without ever climaxing

RIGHT *The woman can stroke her clitoris while her partner thrusts his penis inside her.*

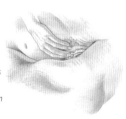

OPPOSITE PAGE *In this position, both partners should be able to orgasm at the same time.*

together during intercourse, but you can change that with the right techniques.

First, you need to find the right position so that the man can thrust into his partner's vagina while still having free access to her clitoris. Ideally, he should lie slightly on one side with the upper leg between both of hers, or on his back with both her legs across him. He can then time his orgasm to coincide with his partner's, as he is in control of both—but he will need clear communication about what she is feeling. Alternatively, she can stroke and rub her own clitoris, but as each partner is now in control of their own climax, communication is even more important if they want to climax together.

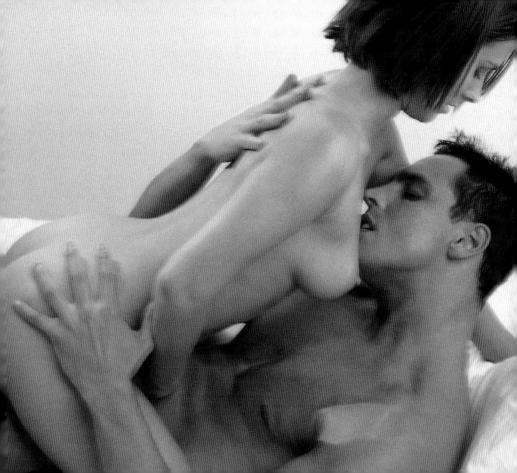

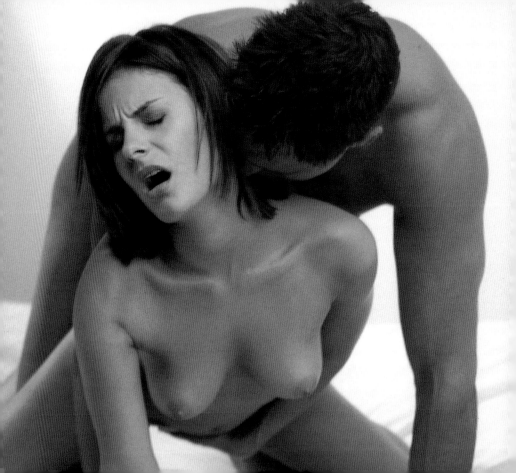

Further Intercourse Techniques

If the position in the previous exercise isn't comfortable or doesn't work for you,
then there are other positions to try. The woman can kneel on the bed and the man can
position himself kneeling behind her. In this position he can enter her from behind
and reach around to stimulate her clitoris.

This position limits the man's ability to thrust sufficiently to achieve his own orgasm, so it is better if the woman reaches down and stimulates the clitoris herself as her partner thrusts inside her. In addition, he can stroke her breasts with one hand to heighten her excitement.

Alternatively, the woman can kneel on all fours with the man kneeling upright behind her, which will enable him to thrust into her easily, but in this case the man will need to be in control of both orgasms. Again, good communication is essential if simultaneous orgasms are to be achieved.

An orgasm in this position will not only be simultaneous but sensational. Ideally, you should come to the plateau stage and then rest for a moment before continuing. Do this as often as you like. It's fun and stimulating to keep being nearly there, then to stop and start again. Good sex shouldn't be rushed; there should be no hurry to achieve orgasm.

The more times you stop at the plateau stage and start again, the more intense and sensational the orgasms will be when you finally decide—together—to let them happen.

LEFT *In this position, the man can thrust into his partner easily and will be able to achieve orgasm. The woman stimulates her clitoris so she can orgasm at the same time.*

The Tail of the Ostrich

In The Perfumed Garden *—an ancient Middle-Eastern sex text—there is a wonderful orgasmic technique delightfully described as "the tail of the ostrich." It is one of the very best sexual techniques if you want to have intercourse. It allows the woman to orgasm by having her clitoris stimulated and allows the man varying levels of penetration.*

THE WOMAN LIES on her back and the man kneels in front of her and lifts her legs until only her neck, the back of her head, and the top of her back are in contact with the bed. He can then enter her from behind, and straighten his back so that he is kneeling upright. She can then cross her ankles behind his head.

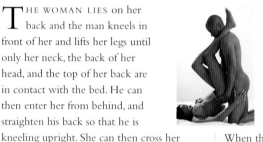

Don't worry, this sounds a lot more difficult than it really is. Once the man has entered his partner, he has both hands free to caress her breasts and stroke her clitoris. In this position, she gets both the benefit of having her partner inside her and of having her clitoris stroked. The man should move gently back and forth and ignore his own orgasm so that she can concentrate on hers.

The advantage of this position is that you can look directly at each other and maintain eye contact. When the man feels that his partner is approaching orgasm, he can thrust as hard as he likes to make sure he comes at the same time. In this position it is really easy.

ABOVE AND RIGHT *In this position the woman can get the best of both worlds; the man can thrust inside her and rub her clitoris.*

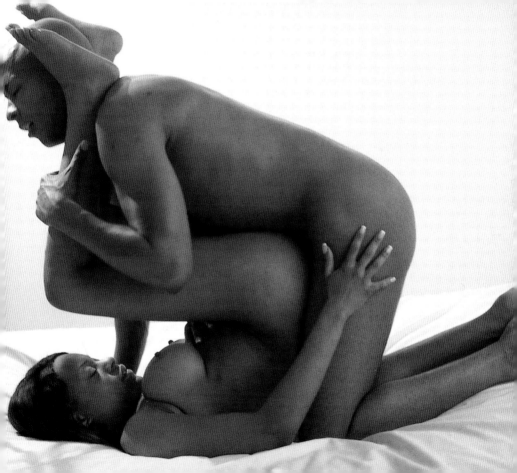

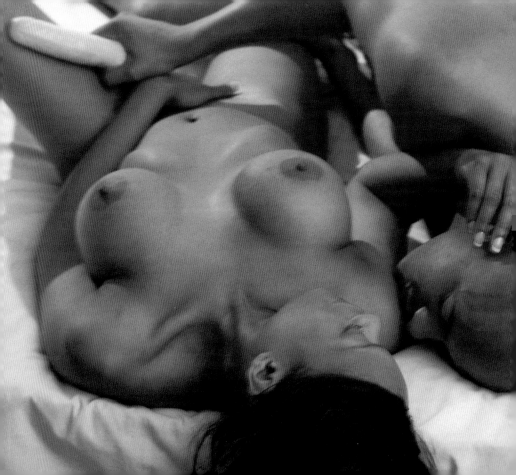

Twice the Pleasure

If you like the idea, you can use a vibrator to enhance your lovemaking. One very good technique is for the man to use a penis-shaped vibrator on his partner while at the same time stimulating her clitoris. If he kneels at her side he can insert the vibrator with one hand and still be able to reach her clitoris with the other.

THE WOMAN WILL also be able to reach her partner's penis to massage it or to even take it into her mouth while she is being masturbated with the vibrator. Some women like sucking on their partner's penis as they orgasm, but it's obviously important not to get too carried away at the moment of climax and to bite instead of suck.

If the man is using the vibrator, he can also use it to stroke his partner's clitoris. In this case he can use his free hand to caress the

LEFT *A vibrator can be used to enhance your lovemaking. While the man is using it to stimulate his partner's clitoris or vagina, she can masturbate or suck his penis.*

entrance to her vagina and can slip one or two fingers into her at the same time, or he can insert his thumb and push downward so he is stimulating her vagina and through to the anal wall as well.

Some vibrators come with an anal prong so the woman can experience both vaginal and rectal stimulation at the same time. The man, still kneeling by her side, can then stroke her clitoris and she can suck on his penis or masturbate her partner. With a little practice it is quite easy for both partners to orgasm simultaneously this way, as long as they keep up the communication about what each of them is feeling.

Women on Top

One of the easiest and best positions in which a couple can enjoy simultaneous orgasms is with the woman on top. If the man lies on his back, she can mount him, allowing her full control over the pace and depth of his penetration. She also has access to her clitoris so she can masturbate to help bring herself to orgasm. At the same time, her partner can also caress her breasts to encourage and stimulate her.

MANY WOMEN find this position very satisfying because of the control it gives them. The woman can slide her vagina up and down the length of the penis with very little effort—a mere tensing of the thighs if she is squatting over her partner. She can even use the head of his penis to stimulate the outer lips of her vagina in order to experience greater pleasure.

A variation on this requires the woman to swivel around so that she is facing away from her partner. This way, his penis will be better

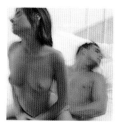

placed to stimulate her G-spot as she slides up and down on him, and she will have good access to both her clitoris and her partner's scrotum, allowing her to stimulate both.

In this position, the woman is in control of both orgasms, so her partner will need to tell her exactly what he is feeling so she can speed up her own orgasm or delay it to keep pace with him.

ABOVE AND RIGHT *In this position, the woman's G-spot is stimulated. She can also touch her clitoris and her partner's scrotum.*

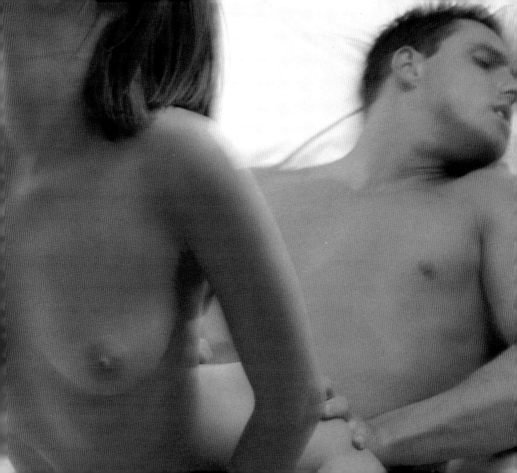

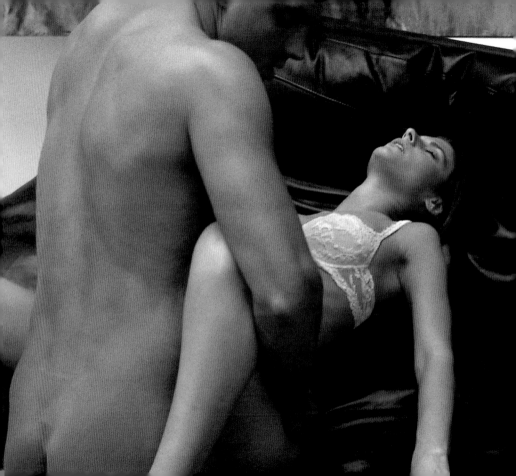

Enjoying Your Lovemaking

The goal of achieving simultaneous orgasms should not interfere with your basic enjoyment of lovemaking. If you become too focused on the end result, you may find yourself losing sight of what it should really be about—having pleasure and fun. There may also be times when you want to make love spontaneously and without any thought of enhancing your orgasms and improving your techniques—a quick bit of passion is all you're after.

AFTER PRACTICING sensational orgasm techniques for a while, however, you will probably find you will want to combine the two. There is one position that seems ideal for this, as it encourages wild passion while still leading to sensational mutual orgasms. In this position the woman should lie on the edge of the bed with her legs reaching down to the floor, although if the bed is the wrong height for her to do this comfortably it is better to

LEFT *In this position the man can thrust easily into the woman and either or both of them can stimulate her clitoris. This position gives good visual stimulation too.*

choose something more suitable, such as a sofa or a low coffee table. The man kneels on the floor and pushes her legs wide apart. He can then enter her, and they both have good access to her clitoris. Either or both of them can stimulate her clitoris to bring her to orgasm, and in this position with his knees on the floor, the man gets good leverage from vigorous thrusting.

This position also allows the man good visual stimulation because he can watch his partner masturbating herself, and he can also caress her breasts. This is also a good position for maintaining eye contact.

The Squeeze Technique

A woman can build up her PC muscle by spending a few minutes each day contracting and relaxing it, as if she were trying to stop and start the flow of urine. This will increase her own orgasmic strength, and she can use the muscle to enhance her partner's orgasms as well. For this next technique she needs to have worked on the muscle for quite a few weeks so it is strong and can be forcefully contracted.

IF THE MAN lies on the bed and the woman crouches above his erect penis, he can enter her without her body touching his anywhere except in the sexual region. She can place her hands on either side of him to support her weight. She should slide her vagina downward until he is completely inside her. Now neither partner should thrust or pump, but should remain absolutely still, maintaining good eye contact and enjoying the warmth and relaxation of this exercise.

The woman can now begin to pump her PC muscle. By contracting and relaxing the muscle along the length of her partner's penis in a strong, rhythmic way, she should be able to bring him to orgasm.

Using the PC muscle to reach an orgasm may not be the quickest means of achieving one, but the orgasm, when it does happen, will be simply sensational for the man. In addition, as the woman will also be incredibly aroused using this method, she will very likely orgasm simultaneously and equally sensationally.

RIGHT *Once the woman has built up her PC muscle, she can forcefully contract and relax it to bring her partner and herself to sensational orgasms.*

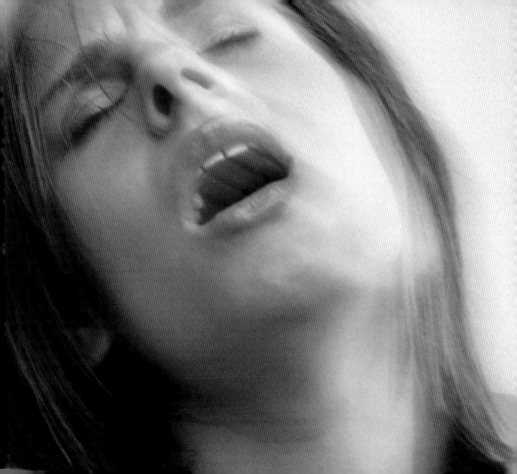

Conclusion, or Climax

You have now explored a lot of techniques for enhancing your orgasms and making them as sensational as possible. I have assumed that you are in a loving, stable, and committed relationship because that is what I know about and what I write about. It is beyond the scope of a book like this to advise on safe sex, contraception, or hygiene, but I assume that you are an adult and know what you are doing. Be safe, but have fun. Improving your lovemaking is one of the greatest skills you can learn. Enjoy your journey.

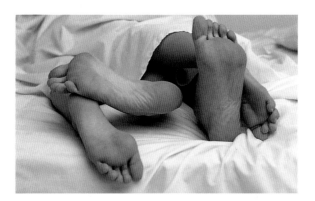